Herbal Medications:

Lessons For Beginners How to Use Homemade Remedies

Table of Contents

Introduction

First I would like to thank and congratulate you on downloading *"Herbal Medicine Made Easy: How to Use Homemade Remedies to Stay Healthy!"* You have made a good choice in deciding to learn more about natural homemade remedies. Natural products will offer you many benefits that synthetic products will not. Using synthetic products filled with artificial ingredients almost always come with often severe side effects. When choosing to use natural herbal remedies you will not have to worry about this. The natural product is the better product by far for many different reasons.

The great thing about natural remedies is that many of the ingredients you can grow in your own garden. There is many medicinal herbs for example that you could grow yourself. This would leave you feeling confident that your own herbs are 100% organically grown and have not been sprayed with any type of harmful chemicals. Not to mention you will save yourself a bundle when you stop purchasing synthetic products and instead use homemade healthy remedies instead. Your body will be much more able to digest natural products and reap the benefits of them compared to synthetic products that your body was not designed to digest. Let us start by taking a look into 'what antibiotics are' in chapter 1.

Chapter 1. What Are Antibiotics?

Many of us at one time or another during our lifetime have taken different forms of antibiotics. We take or took them in the effort to fight off infections. Infections that can come in bacterial or viral forms. The job of antibiotics is to fight off bacterial infections by killing off the bacteria and preventing the bacteria cells from growing. Bacteria is found everywhere. It is in the air we breathe and the water we drink, and it has the ability to cause harmful infections within our bodies. Most bacteria are considered to be harmless, however, there is more variations of bacteria on earth than we are even aware of.

Infections that are caused by bacteria can range from something as simple as an ear infection to more serious infections such as tuberculosis. The job of antibiotics is to kill off the harmful bacteria in our bodies.

The first antibiotics go back to ancient Greeks that used mold based treatments for bacteria. Modern antibiotics were discovered in the 1920's. Alexander Fleming discovered Penicillin in 1928, it was the first modern antibiotic. This discovery paved the way for many other modern antibiotics. Antibiotics such as nitrofurantoin, fluoroquinolon, co-trimoxazole, metronidazole and penicillin all kill the harmful bacteria by blocking it from forming cell walls. These kinds of antibiotics are known as batericidal antibiotics. The antibiotics Tectracyclines, trimethoprim, macrolides, and sulphonamides block the antibiotics from multiplying. These are referred to as bacteriostatic antibiotics.

The modern antibiotics have helped to save millions of lives, but there is still a major downfall to using them. There are various factors involved that have caused these antibiotics to become ineffective over time. There is new bacteria that is referred to as super bugs that are resistant to modern antibiotics. Often the antibiotic is not taken in its full course which results in the bacteria not being completely killed off. Bacteria are basically no different from any other life form in that they will adapt to survive. Bacteria are able to adapt when the antibiotics are not taken in full, making the bacteria stronger to fight against antibiotics. This is a major reason why 'super bugs' have become a major threat to humans.

Due to modern antibiotics becoming less effective more and more people are turning to using natural remedies to improve their health.

Prescription Antibiotics vs. Herbal Antibiotics

When taking modern antibiotics it is crucial to their success that they are taken fully and that the person follows the prescribed treatment. Many people will follow the modern antibiotic treatment until they are feeling better and then do not finish it. They can actually put themselves at risk when stopping treatment and can actually make the infection worse. This is the main reason why bacteria are able to become drug resistant. Not following the treatment through to the end allows the bacteria to build up a resistance to the drug.

There are a number of reasons why the modern antibiotics are becoming less effective such as the compound structure of these antibiotics has effect on their effectiveness. Modern prescription antibiotic are made of one compound and one chemical, they are isolated chemical constituents. This limited compound structure makes it much easier for the bacteria to adapt and defend themselves since they are only fighting against one known compound.

The natural herbal antibiotics have a much more complex structure. Each herbal antibiotic is made up of a variety of different compounds with varying percentages. Take for example the Yarrow plant it has over 120 different compounds that work together to kill off or stop bacteria from growing. It is more effective and less likely that the bacteria will become resistant to it. Due to the fact that there are multiple compounds working together to fight off the bacteria compared to just one compound with modern antibiotics.

Another big plus using herbal antibiotics is that they have no side effects in most cases opposed to the alternative of prescribed antibiotics. Often you will get side effects with prescribed antibiotics from minor to severe, the extreme being death. The only time that prescribed antibiotics should be in use is when there is a life-threatening situation. For minor infections taking a herbal antibiotic you will find this to offer better results, helping to boost your immune system. In time this will help your body to naturally fight off harmful strains of bacteria. Prescription antibiotics can have the opposite affect in that they can cause your body to have difficulty in fighting off bacterial infections.

More and more people find themselves searching for alternative cures such as using herbal antibiotics instead of prescription antibiotics. Many of us will more than likely already have some herbal antibiotics in our homes. As with any medical treatment you are always best to discuss it first with your health care provider. If you are looking into herbal treatments talk to a certified herbalist to get some sound advice on the safest and most effective way you can use herbal antibiotics.

There are some herbal antibiotics that should only be used for a short time period, pregnant women should be cautious of some of the herbal antibiotics.

Chapter 2. Herbal Antibiotics You May Have In Your Kitchen or Garden

You will probably be very surprised as a beginner learning about herbal antibiotics and just how many of them you may already have either in your kitchen or growing in your garden. The best herbal antibiotic are those that are organic, especially when it comes to fighting off infections. Below I have listed some common herbal antibiotics that you may already be using for other reasons such as for their flavor.

1. Onions

Onions are closely related to garlic and come with many special beneficial properties. Packed with numerous antioxidants which includes 25 different flavonols, quercetin, and anthocyanians. The antibacterial properties in onions are prevalent due to the sulfur in onions. Onions are great for fighting against respiratory infections and colds. As I am sure you are already aware there are many variations of onions from yellow to sweet Vidalia to pearl and shallot onions. Each variety of onion offers impressive antibiotic components. The yellow onion offers more sulfuric compounds as well as the most quercetin compared to other varieties of onions. The best results you can gain are from eating raw onions.

2. Turmeric

Turmeric is a very potent antibiotic that offers many healing powers. It has been tested in treatments for cancerous tumors. There is a high level of antioxidants in Turmeric. These high levels make it very effective in fighting off bacteria. Helicobacter plyori is a type of bacteria that grows in the digestive tract that attacks the stomach lining and can cause ulcers in the stomach and small intestine. The curcumin found in Turmeric plays a vital role in fighting against this particular bacteria. There is many different ways that we can consume Turmeric, from a paste form to mixing it in warm milk. It can help treat respiratory infections and prevent a number of bacterial infections. A good way to help prevent these kinds of health issues is to take a teaspoon of Turmeric a day or supplement.

3. Garlic

Garlic has been used as a form of medicine for centuries throughout human history. Garlic is a very effective antibiotic due to its sulphur compound, antibacterial, antioxidant and also its anti-hypertensive components. Including garlic as part of your daily diet is accompanied with a long list of benefits. Garlic is well known in helping to reduce blood pressure, improve the body's immune system and is a powerful antibiotic. There is numerous agents that are antiviral, antibacterial, antifungal that are found in garlic.

Garlic is one of the most affordable herbal antibiotics that you can find in most if not all grocery stores. It can help to fight off flu infections, colds, tooth infections and even some symptoms of the AIDS virus have shown to become reduced with the consumption of garlic. It is often used in fighting off digestive and urinary tract infections. Garlic is such a powerful antibiotic largely due to the phytochemical allicin found in it, which is highly effective in fighting against the MRSA superbug.

The most potent way to eat garlic is raw, but this could cause you to have bad breath and body odor. It comes in other forms such as capsules and oils. If you consume 2-4 cloves of garlic a day this can help kill off unwanted bacteria. You can do this by adding it to your salads or to your morning smoothie or soup. You may like to consume it by making a garlic tea by boiling the cloves in water for a few minutes.

4. Cinnamon

Cinnamon is well known for its ability to lower blood sugars as well as contains anti-inflammatory properties. It also offers a number of antibiotic properties as well. It has antiviral, antifungal, and antimicrobial properties, making it very effective in fighting off a wide variety of infections. Cinnamon is a good at helping to treat a number of infections, including yeast infection and is even connected to helping kill off the deadly E.coli bacteria.

One of the best ways to consume cinnamon is by boiling it in some water and sipping on it like a cup of tea. You can drink this beverage hot or cold, several times a day. Add some honey to it to make an even more potent antibiotic with some added sweetness in the flavor.

5. *Honey*

Manuka and New Zealand honey have both been used in treating wounds due to their powerful antibacterial and anti-inflammatory properties. Manuka honey contains methylgyoxal which is a very effective antibacterial compound. It is found in high doses in Manuka honey. This herbal antibiotic has been shown to be good for long term use as it takes people a long time to build up a resistance to it. Manuka honey has been shown to very effective in fighting against over 200 different strains of bacteria and diseases.

Many people like to combine their Manuka honey in a herbal to gain the combine benefits of these as a herbal antibiotic. Do not cook honey as it could lead to the release of toxins.

6. *Horseradish*

Horseradish is packed with beneficial compounds that can help in the promotion of blood circulation and when it is broken down inside the stomach it releases antibiotic properties.

Horseradish works as a good antibiotic against infections such as urinary tract infections, bronchitis, and kidney stones. The best way to consume horseradish is raw.

7. *Curry Powder*

Curry powder makes a great antibiotic for a number of reasons. The most common spices found in curry powder are: ginger, turmeric, and coriander. Each of these individual spices have antibacterial properties that help ward off infections and diseases. When mixed in curry powder you are getting a combined mix of powerful antibacterial compounds. Together this mix can help to kill a wide range of bacterial infections.

8. *Baking Soda*

Baking soda helps to regulate the pH balance. It helps in the treatment of skin infections, respiratory and intestinal infections. You can use baking soda in a number of ways in order to treat numerous kinds of infections. You can add a cup of baking soda to your bath water and soak in it for 20 minutes to help alleviate skin infections. You may also choose to make a paste by adding a few drops of water and adding it directly on the infected area. To help with stomach upset you can mix half a teaspoon into a glass of water and drink it.

9. Ginger

Ginger has been used for thousands of years to treat digestive problems. Ginger is great in helping to prevent food borne pathogens such as salmonella and listeria from attacking your body. Ginger is also good in treating allergies, nausea, colic, motion sickness and for pain relief. You can take ginger raw, tea, oil, tincture or in tablet form.

10. Cranberry Juice

Drinking 100% pure organic cranberry juice is great for helping to treat vaginal infections and urinary tract infections. You need to use 100% pure unsweetened cranberry juice so that you will gain use of the vital compounds that make it an effective antibiotic.

11. Lemon

Lemon works well in treating respiratory infections, it helps to break down mucus in the respiratory tract. When the mucus is removed the bacteria will be removed with it.

12. Cardamom

This is a very powerful spice that has been used in Chinese and Indian medicines for thousands of years. The antimicrobial properties that cardamom contains help to fight against a number of health issues such as blood pressure and gastrointestinal diseases. It also can help to treat gum disease and tooth infections. It is well known in helping the body to rid itself of harmful toxins and bacteria.

Chapter 3. Herbal Teas, Oils, Syrups, Tinctures, & Salves

If you are preparing herbal medicines at home you will probably apply them using teas, oils, tinctures, and salves. When preparing them at home you will know 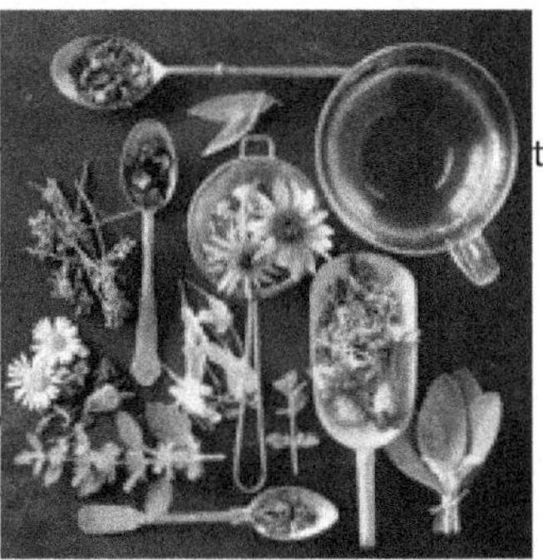 t h e strength of the product you are preparing, when purchasing products you do not always know the quantities of healing herbs.   The FDA has even determined that commercial preparations may have no herbs in them at all, instead they may contain an imitation product.

Teas

You can make teas using dried herbs, allowing them to steep in hot water for at least five minutes. This will allow the tea to extract the essence of the herb. Strain the tea using a tea strainer to remove any stems or seeds. You can drink these teas hot or cold. Add in some honey to sweeten them if you wish.

Syrups

You can make syrups from the concentrated extracts of herbs. Often people will choose to add some honey to syrups to help improve the taste of them.   Syrups work well in helping to relieve sore throats and coughs.

To Prepare Syrups:

- 2 cups of dried herbs

- 4 cups of cold water

- honey

- 1 cinnamon stick

Combine the cinnamon stick, herbs and cold water and bring these to a boil over medium heat in a pot. When it begins to boil reduce heat to a simmer for 45 minutes. Strain mix through cheesecloth while liquid is warm. Measure the liquid and add in the same amount of honey. Stir in the honey until it is completely dissolved over low heat. Do not allow the mix to boil. Add mix to dark glass bottle.

Oils
Solar Method of Oil Preparation:

- Place your dried herbs into a sterilized glass jar. The herbs can be whole, crushed, ground or chopped. Cover the herbs with a carrier oil such as extra virgin olive oil. Leave a gap of about 2-inches at top of bottle. This will allow space for swelling of herbs.

- Cape the bottle and place in a southern facing window. You can cover with paper bag so that it is not getting direct sunlight.

- Daily shake and turn the bottle.

- If oil is absorbed by the herbs add in more oil.

- Infuse the mix for 6 weeks, then strain through cheesecloth to remove plant stems etc.

- Bottle into sterilized amber glass bottles.

- Add in vitamin E as this will help prolong the mixes shelf life.

- It should have a shelf life of at least 1 year, store in cool, dark place.

Crock Pot Method of Oil Preparation:

- Place your herb combination within your crock pot. Add in extra virgin olive oil, to cover the herbs. Leave head room of about 2-inches to allow herbs to swell.

- Leave on low in crock pot for 72 hours, adding oil if necessary.

- Slowly stir the ingredients.

- Turn off the heat source and allow the mix to cool.

- Strain mix through cheesecloth, bottle in sterilized bottles.

- Store up to one year in cool dark place.

- Add in Vitamin E oil to prolong shelf life.

Tinctures and Liquid Extracts

In the process of making tinctures the herbal stems and leaves are used along with seeds, dissolved in water, alcohol or glycerol. They usually consist of a concentration of 1:5 or 1:10. This means one part herb compound is mixed together with either 5 or 10 parts liquid. Liquid extracts are stronger than tinctures and are usually prepared with 1:1 concentration.

Making Tinctures & Extracts:

Fresh Herbs
- Using fresh herbs finely chop them

- Fill a jar 2/3 with herbs or 1/2 with roots

- Cover completely with alcohol

Dried Herbs
- Fincly chop herbs

- Fill a jar 3/4 with herbs or 1/3 of roots.

- The herbs and roots will absorb alcohol and they will expand by half of their size.

- Cover the herbs with alcohol.

Alcohol Additives
- Use 40-50% use 80-90 proof vodka

- 70% use 1/2 vodka and 1/2 pure grain alcohol, 190 proof.

- 95% use 190 pure grain alcohol.

Extraction Bottling

Allow your bottle preparation to meld for at least six weeks. Shake the bottle every day and add alcohol as it is absorbed. The herbs should always be covered by alcohol to prohibit bacteria and mold. After the six weeks strain through cheesecloth. Label mixture. Store in a cool, dark area. Tinctures can last indefinitely.

Salves

Salves are made from infused oils with beeswax added for firming.

- Start with 8 ounces of infused oil preparation

- Add 1 ounce of beeswax into a double broiler or crock pot.

- Heat until the beeswax has melted.

- Add in a few drops of vitamin E oil, 10 drops of an essential oil such as lavender.

- Pour mixture into a tin or shallow glass to re-solidify, storing in cool location, this can last up to 3 years.

Dry Extracts

Dry extracts are commercially prepared herbs that are sold at all kinds of major retailers. They are bottled and sold in pills, capsules, and other forms by an outside agent.

Chapter 4. Medicinal Herbal Recipes and Remedies

In this chapter you will discover recipes and remedies that can help to get you feeling healthy again. These are remedies that will help you to improve your health. Make sure to give the remedies time to take effect before you decide to start increasing the dosage.

1. Bee Sting:

Using a bit of lavender essential oil will help neutralize the venom from a bee sting. After you have neutralized the venom add a bit of toothpaste to help relieve the pain.

2. Infections:

Hot and cold compresses work well. You can make a hot compress to treat backache, toothache, or other pains by adding essential oil to some hot water and then dipping cloth into water and applying to infected area. Make a cold compress for areas such as sprains or strains by adding essential oil to ice water before placing on affected area.

3. Viruses and cold:

Ginger is a great natural treatment to use for colds and viruses. You can make a tea using fresh ginger, with a little honey and a dash of cayenne pepper.

4. Acid reflux:

Have a cup of herbal tea after each meal to help with acid related or upset stomach. Some good teas to try for this are chamomile, ginger, mint.

5. Poison ivy:

Make a salve using Jewelweed.

Ingredients:

- 1/4 cup of herb

- 1/4 of chamomile dried flowers or Siberian elm bark

- olive oil

- 2 ounces of beeswax that is melted

Directions:

Add in olive oil to about 1/4 inch up on the side of dish, cover and bake in oven at low setting for a couple of hours. Allow mix to cool then press down on baking sheet. Reheat adding 2 ounces of beeswax that is melted. Allow mix to cool and apply to affected area.

6. Rashes:

Using a cotton ball apply Echinea tincture to a rash.

7. Homemade lip balm:

Using this lip balm is a great way to help protect your lips in the cold weather.

Ingredients:

Oil Mixture

- 4 ounces of a carrier oil, such as coconut oil

- cut and sifted alkanet root (1 tablespoon)

- half a cup of evergreen tree needles

Essential Oil Mixture:

- 1 ounce of Shea butter

- 1 1/2 ounces of beeswax

- 20 drops each of peppermint and Douglas fir essential oils

- 1/2 teaspoon vitamin E oil

- 1/4 teaspoon rosemary

Directions:

Heat the oil mixture ingredients in a double broiler until mix is warm to the touch. Allow to cool for a couple of hours. Heat again and repeat in 24 hours. Once this process is complete strain the oil mixture to remove plant parts. Next add essential oil mixture ingredients into the double broiler and heat on low until all is melted. Stir well add in oil mixture and stir. Use a funnel to pour the mixture into small lip balm containers. It will pour easily then it will solidify in lip balm containers.

8. Rose Petal Honey

Fill a small glass jar with fresh rose petals, pour honey over petals. This will make a great topical treatment for pain.

9. Self-heal Skin Serum
Ingredients:

- 5 ounces of jojoba oil

- 4 ounces of argon oil

- 1 ounce pomegranate oil

- 1/2 an ounce of self-heal herb

- 1 teaspoon of rosemary

- 20 drops neroli essential oil

- 3 drops blue chamomile essential oil

- 6 drops lavender essential oil

Directions:

In a double broiler add in jojoba, argon, pomegranate oils along with self-heal herb. Warm the mixture until it is warm to the touch. Remove and allow to sit for awhile then reheat but do not overheat mix. Maintain the heat for 24 hours, remove from heat and place in blender on high. Strain the mixture then add in the remaining ingredients. Mix well then store in an airtight container.

10. Arnica Ointment
Ingredients:

- 3/4 of an ounce of Shea butter

- 3/4 of an ounce of coconut oil

- 3/4 of an ounce of beeswax

- 3/4 cup Arnica and St. John's wort oil mixture

- 2/3 cup helichrysum

- 25 drops lavender essential oil

Directions:

Add the beeswax, Shea butter, coconut oil into double broiler and heat on low until all is melted. Remove from heat and add in the rest of ingredients mix. Add to a blender and slowly blend. Store in small airtight containers.

11. Chamomile & Olive Massage Oil
This is a great herbal recipe that can help your muscles to relax and will also help lubricate your skin.

Ingredients:

- 12 ounces olive oil

- 1 ounce chamomile flowers

Directions:

Place your chamomile flowers into mortar and pestle and lightly bruise them. Mix the chamomile flowers with olive oil in glass bowl. Pour mix into glass jar and allow to sit in sun for several days. Each day make sure to give the mix a swirl. On the seventh day strain mix through cheesecloth. Pour mix into dark glass bottles for storage, store in cool dark place.

12. Garlic Fungal Cream

Athlete's foot, jock itch, Candida, Nail fungus etc. Garlic works as a wonderful antifungal and is highly effective at treating any type of fungal infection.

Ingredients:

- 2 cloves of garlic

- olive oil

Directions:

Crush your cloves of garlic. Add in a few drops of olive oil to form a paste. Apply to the affected area and leave on for 30 minutes. Wash the area with warm water and dry. Do this procedure 2 times daily. If you have a vaginal fungus infection just wrap a piece of garlic in some gauze and place on vagina area for 30 minutes. Do this once a day for a several day period. Also add garlic to your foods to help speed up fungal treatment.

13. Catnip & Chamomile Sleepy Tincture

This is a natural herbal tincture that will help your body to relax so it can ease into sleep.

Ingredients:

- 4 tablespoons of yarrow flowers, dried

- 2 tablespoons of Stevia leaf, dried

- 2 tablespoons of mint leaves, dried

- 4 tablespoons chamomile flowers

- 4 tablespoons catnip, dried

- 4 tablespoons of oat straw, dried

- 2 tablespoons hops flowers, dried

- boiling water

- 4 cups 80 proof or stronger vodka

Directions:

Put all of the herbs into 2 glass jars, split mix in half. Pour boiling water so that it just covers the herbs. Mix well. Top off with vodka. Close using airtight lid. Store in dark, cool place for 6 to 8 weeks. Shake contents in jars daily. After 6-8 weeks strain out the herbs. Store in small glass jars and use as you need it. Dose is 2-3 droppers full for adults and 1 dropper for kids over 2 years of age.

14. *Healthy Heart Tonic*

This tincture is very powerful in helping to boost your energy. This ginseng and hawthorn tincture will have your heart pumping in no time. If you take prescribed heart medication talk to your physician before using this treatment.

Ingredients:

- 1 part hawthorn

- 1 part ginseng

- 2 parts olive leaf

Directions:

Mix your ingredients in a bowl. Fill 00 capsules. Start taking one capsule a day or increase to two a day until you get the desired effect.

15. *Honey & Mullein Cough Syrup*
Ingredients:

- 2/3 ounce mullein

- 2/3 ounce rosehip

- 2/3 ounce coltsfoot

- 4 ounces honey

Directions:

Crush the rosehip until they are course. Place them into saucepan along with coltsfoot and mullein. Add in 2 cups water and stir. Bring mix to a boil. Boil until there is half the liquid, this will take about 20 minutes. Let it cool. Pour through cheesecloth. Pour back into saucepan and reheat, but do not let it boil. Add in honey and stir. Store in brown glass bottles with airtight lids. The shelf life for this cough syrup is one month.

16. *Goldenseal Respiratory Treatment*
You can use this remedy to treat colds, asthma, flu congestion, coughs and other respiratory ailments.

Ingredients:

- 1 part mullein

- 3 parts ephedra

- 1 part Goldenseal

- 1 part coltsfoot

- 1 part comfrey

- 1 part marshmallow

- 1 part lobelia

- 1 part cayenne

Directions:

Grind herbs finely mix ingredients well then place into 00 capsules and take 1-2 capsules 2-3 times a day until you are feeling better.

17. Eucalyptus Liniment
Ingredients:

- 1 ounce of lobelia

- 24 ounces rubbing alcohol or vodka

- 1 1/2 ounces of eucalyptus

- 1/2 ounce of cayenne

Directions:

Take a quart jar and wash it well, add in herbs. Pour 16 ounces rubbing alcohol into jar and seal tight. Label jar for external use only. Shake up the mix. Place in dark cool place for at least 1 week. Strain the herbs using a cheesecloth, press herbs while doing this. Pour into dark bottles for storage and label. Rub into skin when applying it a few times.

Conclusion

I hope that you and your loved ones will enjoy using the tips and suggestions I offer in my book in regards to learning a bit more about medicinal herbs and their uses and how you can grow them yourself and make your very own homemade herbal remedies. I myself love using my own organically grown herbs from my boxed garden to make all kinds of great remedies and recipes with. I am sure you too will find the same kind of pleasure when you make your first homemade remedy using your own homegrown medicinal herbs!

I just want to thank you once again for downloading my book, I cannot express to you how much your support of my work means to me. I would love to read a review by you in Amazon of my book! Take care and happy growing and preparing your own medicinal herbs!